THE CORTISOL DETOX
DIET PLAN

A Step-by-Step Guide to Regaining Control Over
Stress, Anxiety, and Hormonal Imbalances

Grace Mitchell

Table of Content

INTRODUCTION

Welcome to a journey towards a healthier, calmer you. If you've picked up this book, chances are you're ready to take back control—not just of your diet, but of your life. Stress, anxiety, and hormonal imbalances may have brought you here, but through the pages of this guide, you'll find the pathway to renewal and balance. Let's embark on this transformative journey together.

What is Cortisol?

Cortisol, often referred to as the "stress hormone," is essential for helping your body deal with stressful situations. Produced by your adrenal glands, this hormone helps regulate blood pressure, reduce inflammation, and assist in the metabolism of fats, carbohydrates, and proteins. However, while cortisol is vital for survival, its overproduction can be detrimental.

Understanding the Impact of Cortisol on Your Health

The effects of cortisol extend far beyond the immediate response to stress. When your cortisol levels remain chronically high, it can lead to a host of health issues—weight gain, high blood pressure, sleep disturbances, and a weakened immune system, to name a few. Perhaps more critically, it can also disrupt your other hormonal balances, leading to a cascade of health problems that can feel overwhelming.

The Importance of Managing Cortisol Levels

Balancing your cortisol is not just about improving your physical health—it's about reclaiming your life from the clutches of stress and anxiety. Managing cortisol levels can enhance your mood, boost your energy levels, and help you regain a restful night's sleep. It is a crucial step toward not only living longer but living better.

How to Use This Book

This book is designed as a step-by-step guide to detoxing your body from excess cortisol through thoughtful diet choices, lifestyle changes, and emotional well-being practices. Each chapter builds on the last, providing you with a comprehensive plan that starts at understanding the basics of cortisol and leads you through detailed, practical strategies for achieving and maintaining balance.

From meal plans and recipes to stress-reduction techniques and mindfulness exercises, we'll cover all the tools you need to reduce your cortisol levels and enhance your overall health. Follow the chapters sequentially to build a strong foundation of knowledge, and refer back to specific sections as needed to reinforce particular aspects of your detox plan.

You are not alone on this journey. With every page, you'll gain more insights and tools to help you manage stress, balance your hormones, and restore your body to its natural, intended rhythm. Let's begin this important work together.

THE SCIENCE BEHIND THE CORTISOL DETOX DIET PLAN

In this chapter, we delve into the intricate relationship between cortisol and your overall well-being. Understanding the dual impact of cortisol on both body and mind is crucial for appreciating why a detox plan focused on this hormone can be profoundly transformative. We will also explore the interconnectedness of stress, anxiety, and hormonal balance, supported by research that underscores the effectiveness of dietary interventions in managing cortisol levels.

How Cortisol Affects Your Body and Mind

Cortisol is not just a biological response to stress; it's a powerful hormone that plays multiple roles across various bodily functions. In short bursts, cortisol can provide the necessary energy boost required to handle emergencies and meet daily challenges. However, when cortisol levels remain high over an extended period, the effects can be damaging.

Physically, excessive cortisol can lead to weight gain, particularly around the stomach, high blood pressure, and osteoporosis. It can disrupt sleep, lower immune function, and increase the risk of chronic diseases such as type 2 diabetes and heart disease.

Mentally, high cortisol impairs cognitive functions such as memory and concentration and exacerbates symptoms of mental health disorders, including anxiety and depression. It creates a vicious cycle where stress raises cortisol levels, which in turn increase feelings of anxiety and unrest, further elevating stress and cortisol.

The Connection Between Anxiety, Stress, and Hormones

Stress and anxiety are not just emotional states; they have a profound effect on the hormonal milieu of the body. When you're stressed, your body's fight or flight response is triggered, leading to a surge of adrenaline and cortisol. This response is supposed to subside once the immediate threat passes.

However, persistent stress means cortisol levels stay elevated, disrupting not only cortisol balance but also affecting other hormones like insulin, sex hormones, and neurotransmitters.

This hormonal imbalance can exacerbate the physical symptoms of stress and lead to further anxiety and depression, creating a feedback loop that can be difficult to break without intervention.

Research/Studies Supporting the Effectiveness of a Cortisol Detox Diet

Emerging research highlights the role of diet in modulating cortisol levels and mitigating the effects of stress. Studies indicate that certain foods can either provoke or dampen the body's cortisol response. For instance, foods rich in vitamin C, omega-3 fatty acids, and magnesium have been shown to lower cortisol levels.

A pivotal study published in the Journal of Clinical Endocrinology & Metabolism found that high dietary glycemic index increases the production of cortisol by the adrenal glands, suggesting that a low-glycemic diet might aid in managing cortisol levels. Moreover, clinical trials have shown that adapting meal frequency and timing can also play a significant role in stabilizing cortisol throughout the day.

Furthermore, integrating anti-inflammatory foods into one's diet not only assists in reducing the production of cortisol but also helps in repairing the body damaged by long-term exposure to high cortisol levels, thereby affirmatively supporting the theory behind the Cortisol Detox Diet.

In conclusion, the science underlying the Cortisol Detox Diet Plan is both compelling and empowering. As we move forward in this book, you will learn how to apply this knowledge through dietary changes, lifestyle adjustments, and stress management techniques to effectively reduce cortisol levels and enhance your overall health.

ASSESSING YOUR CORTISOL LEVELS

Recognizing the signs of cortisol imbalance and understanding how to accurately measure and interpret your levels are the first crucial steps toward recovery. This chapter guides you through the symptoms to watch for, the tests available, and how to comprehend what your results mean for your health. Here, you'll gain the knowledge you need to take proactive steps toward regaining your balance and vitality.

Identifying Symptoms of High Cortisol Levels

Cortisol affects various systems in your body, and therefore, its symptoms can be diverse and sometimes subtle. You might feel as though you're just not your best self, and perhaps you've noticed some changes that concern you. Common signs of high cortisol levels include:

- Persistent fatigue despite getting enough sleep, leaving you feeling drained and exhausted.

- Weight gain, especially around the abdomen and face, which can be sudden and difficult to control.

- Mood swings that feel uncontrollable and frequent feelings of anxiety or depression.

- Difficulty concentrating or feelings of mental fog that hinder your daily activities.

- Increased thirst and frequency of urination, which can disrupt your daily life.

- Sleep disturbances, where you find it hard to fall or stay asleep despite feeling tired.

- Weakened immune response, leading to more frequent infections or prolonged recovery times.

If you notice these symptoms, it might be time to explore further with professional guidance to see if cortisol is a contributing factor.

Diagnostic Tests for Measuring Cortisol Levels

Fortunately, assessing your cortisol levels can be done with accuracy through several types of diagnostic tests. The most common include:

- **Saliva test:** This test measures your cortisol levels at different times of the day and is widely used due to its convenience. It can be done at home using a kit and then sent to a lab for analysis.

- **Blood test:** Often conducted in the morning when cortisol levels should be naturally higher, this test provides a snapshot of how your adrenal glands are functioning.

- **Urine test:** This 24-hour test gives a broader picture of cortisol production throughout a day. You'll collect all your urine in a special container over a 24-hour period for analysis.

Each of these tests has its advantages, and your healthcare provider can help determine which is best for your specific situation.

Understanding the Results and Interpreting Your Cortisol Profile

Once your results are in, the next step is to understand what they mean. Interpreting these results can be complex because normal cortisol levels can vary widely among individuals. Generally, higher than normal levels may indicate that your body is under continuous stress, which is negatively impacting your health.

Your doctor can help you understand your specific cortisol profile in the context of your symptoms and medical history. They will look at:

- **Daily patterns:** Normally, cortisol levels peak in the morning and decline throughout the day. Abnormal patterns, such as elevated cortisol at night, can disrupt sleep and impact overall health.

- **Response to stress:** How your cortisol levels change in response to stress can also provide insights into your adrenal health and stress management needs.

THE PRINCIPLES OF THE CORTISOL DETOX DIET PLAN

Embarking on the Cortisol Detox Diet Plan involves understanding and implementing specific dietary principles, selecting the right foods, and integrating lifestyle modifications that help manage cortisol levels effectively. This chapter lays out a clear, detailed pathway to help you regulate your body's cortisol production, leading to improved health and vitality.

Nutrients That Help Regulate Cortisol Levels

Regulating cortisol levels can be significantly influenced by your diet, particularly through the intake of specific nutrients that help manage this crucial stress hormone. Here are some key nutrients known to help regulate cortisol levels:

Vitamin C: This vitamin is essential for reducing cortisol levels in the body, especially during times of stress. It helps to modulate the cortisol response, aiding in quicker recovery from stressful situations. Good sources of Vitamin C include citrus fruits, strawberries, bell peppers, and broccoli.

Omega-3 Fatty Acids: These essential fats have powerful anti-inflammatory properties and can help reduce the production of cortisol during stressful times. They are found in high concentrations in fatty fish like salmon, mackerel, and sardines, as well as in flaxseeds, chia seeds, and walnuts.

Magnesium: Magnesium has been referred to as the relaxation mineral because it plays a role in deactivating adrenaline and can help calm the nervous system, thereby reducing cortisol levels. Foods rich in magnesium include leafy green vegetables (like spinach and Swiss chard), nuts, seeds, and whole grains.

Phosphatidylserine: This phospholipid, found in cell membranes, is thought to play a role in reducing cortisol when under stress. It can be taken as a supplement, and is also found in foods like soybeans, egg yolks, and white beans.

B Vitamins: Particularly vitamins B5 (pantothenic acid), B6, and B12, have been found to support adrenal function, help manage stress, and regulate cortisol levels. B5 is essential for the production of adrenal hormones. B6 aids in the production of serotonin, which can help manage stress, and B12 supports energy production. Foods rich in B vitamins include whole grains, meats, eggs, nuts, and avocados.

Zinc: Zinc plays a significant role in modulating the brain and body's response to stress. It can help control cortisol levels and support brain health. Foods high in zinc include beef, oysters, pumpkin seeds, and lentils.

L-Theanine: An amino acid found primarily in tea leaves, L-Theanine promotes relaxation without drowsiness. It can mitigate the body's cortisol response to physical and mental stress.

Ashwagandha: Though not a nutrient but a herb, Ashwagandha is known for its adaptogenic properties, helping the body to manage stress and reduce cortisol levels.

Foods to Include for Optimal Cortisol Regulation

To help regulate cortisol levels effectively through your diet, it's beneficial to focus on foods that nourish and calm your body. Here are several types of foods recommended to include in your diet for optimal cortisol regulation:

1. **Whole Grains:** Consuming whole grains like oats, quinoa, brown rice, and barley can help maintain stable blood sugar levels and thus reduce cortisol spikes. They provide a steady source of energy throughout the day without the sharp insulin spikes associated with refined carbs.

2. **Leafy Greens and Vegetables:** Vegetables, especially leafy greens like spinach, kale, and Swiss chard, are rich in vitamins and minerals such as magnesium and antioxidants that support adrenal health and help reduce stress-induced damage in the body.

3. **Fatty Fish:** Salmon, mackerel, sardines, and trout are high in omega-3 fatty acids, which are known for their anti-inflammatory properties and ability to help reduce cortisol levels.

4. **Citrus Fruits and Berries:** Fruits like oranges, grapefruits, lemons, and berries are rich in vitamin C, a nutrient that can help lower cortisol and support adrenal function.

5. **Nuts and Seeds:** Almonds, walnuts, flaxseeds, and chia seeds provide healthy fats, magnesium, and zinc, all of which help in controlling cortisol levels and supporting overall health.

6. **Legumes:** Beans, lentils, and chickpeas are great sources of protein and fiber, which help to stabilize blood sugar levels, preventing cortisol spikes.

7. **Fermented Foods:** Foods like yogurt, kefir, sauerkraut, and kimchi are rich in probiotics, which support gut

health. A healthy gut can improve your overall health and resilience to stress.

8. **Herbal Teas:** Certain herbal teas like green tea, ashwagandha tea, and holy basil (tulsi) tea contain compounds that can help reduce stress and cortisol levels. L-theanine in green tea, for example, promotes relaxation and helps in mitigating stress responses.

9. **Avocados:** Rich in B vitamins and monounsaturated fats, avocados are excellent for adrenal health. B vitamins are crucial for healthy brain function and combating stress, while healthy fats provide sustained energy.

10. **Dark Chocolate:** High in flavonoids, dark chocolate (at least 70% cocoa) can reduce cortisol and has been shown to boost mood. However, it should be consumed in moderation due to its calorie content.

Foods to Avoid to Minimize Cortisol Spikes

To minimize cortisol spikes and better manage stress, it's important to be mindful of certain foods and substances that can exacerbate cortisol production. Here are some foods and beverages you might consider avoiding or reducing in your diet:

Caffeine: High doses of caffeine found in coffee, tea, energy drinks, and some sodas can increase cortisol levels. If you're sensitive to caffeine or experience anxiety after consuming it, consider cutting back or choosing caffeine-free alternatives.

Sugar and High-Glycemic Carbohydrates: Sugary snacks, desserts, and drinks, as well as refined carbohydrates like white bread and pastries, can cause rapid spikes in blood sugar and insulin levels, leading to increased cortisol. Opt for low-glycemic, whole food options instead.

Processed Foods: Many processed foods contain high levels of sugar, unhealthy fats, and additives—all of which can affect cortisol levels. Processed meats, canned foods, and prepackaged snacks typically fall into this category.

Trans Fats: Found in some margarines, snack foods, and baked goods, trans fats can promote inflammation and may affect cortisol levels. Check labels for hydrogenated oils and avoid foods that contain them.

Alcohol: While moderate alcohol consumption may have some health benefits, excessive intake can disrupt the balance of the body's systems, including hormonal levels like cortisol. Alcohol can also interfere with sleep, further impacting cortisol production.

Fried Foods: Besides being high in trans fats and calories, fried foods are harder to digest and can cause discomfort and stress to your digestive system, potentially raising cortisol levels.

Artificial Sweeteners: Some studies suggest that artificial sweeteners like aspartame may trigger insulin release and possibly cortisol responses, just like sugar. Opt for natural sweeteners in moderation, such as honey or maple syrup.

Dairy Products: In some individuals, especially those with a sensitivity or intolerance to lactose or dairy proteins, dairy products can cause inflammation and possibly elevate cortisol levels. Monitor how your body responds to dairy and consider reducing intake if necessary.

Highly Spicy and Acidic Foods: For some people, spicy and acidic foods can cause gastrointestinal irritation, which can be a stressor leading to increased cortisol levels.

Gluten: For individuals with celiac disease or gluten sensitivity, consuming gluten can trigger an immune response and increase stress and inflammation, thus potentially raising cortisol levels.

Creating a Personalized Cortisol Detox Meal Plan

Creating a personalized Cortisol Detox Meal Plan is a vital step towards managing your stress levels and improving your overall health. This plan will focus on incorporating foods that help lower cortisol and excluding those that might trigger its production. Here's a step-by-step guide to creating your meal plan:

Step 1: Evaluate Your Current Diet

Begin by keeping a food diary for a week. Record everything you eat and drink, noting the times of your meals and how you feel afterward. This will help you identify any habits that may be contributing to cortisol spikes, such as consuming high-sugar snacks or caffeine at times of day when stress peaks.

Step 2: Identify Foods to Include and Avoid

Based on the principles discussed earlier about foods that regulate cortisol and those that cause spikes, make a list of foods to focus on and those to reduce or eliminate. For instance, increase your intake of whole grains, lean proteins, fruits and vegetables, and healthy fats. Plan to reduce caffeine, sugar, processed foods, and high-glycemic carbs.

Step 3: Plan Your Meals

Create a meal plan that incorporates the beneficial foods into every meal and snack. Aim for balance in macronutrients (carbohydrates, proteins, and fats) to ensure sustained energy levels throughout the day. Here's a simple framework:

- **Breakfast:** Start with a good source of protein and fiber to stabilize blood sugar levels from the start. For example, an omelet with spinach and mushrooms, or oatmeal topped with nuts and berries.
- **Lunch:** Focus on lean protein and plenty of vegetables. A salad with grilled chicken, mixed greens, avocado, nuts, and a vinaigrette, or a vegetable stir-fry with tofu or fish can be great options.
- **Dinner:** Similar to lunch, emphasize proteins and vegetables. Try something like baked salmon with quinoa and steamed broccoli, or a turkey and vegetable stew.

- **Snacks:** Choose snacks that include protein and healthy fats to keep energy levels stable. Examples include yogurt with flaxseeds, an apple with almond butter, or a small handful of mixed nuts.

Step 4: Incorporate Stress-Reducing Techniques

Plan specific times in your schedule for stress-reduction activities. This could be morning meditation, yoga sessions, or evening walks. Regular physical activity not only helps reduce cortisol levels directly but also improves your overall health.

Step 5: Adjust as Needed

Your cortisol detox plan should be flexible. Pay attention to how your body reacts to different foods and activities. If you notice that certain foods or patterns aren't working for you, adjust your plan accordingly. This could mean swapping out certain foods, changing meal times, or trying different stress-reduction techniques.

Step 6: Stay Hydrated

Don't forget to drink plenty of water throughout the day. Hydration is crucial for all bodily functions, including hormone production and stress management.

Step 7: Review and Reflect

After a few weeks on your meal plan, review your food diary and any changes in how you feel. Are your stress levels lower? Do you have more energy? Keep what works and tweak what doesn't to refine your plan over time.

Incorporating Exercise and Stress-Reducing Techniques into Your Routine

Incorporating exercise and stress-reducing techniques into your daily routine is essential for effectively managing cortisol levels and improving your overall well-being. Exercise not only helps reduce cortisol directly but also enhances mood and energy levels. Similarly, stress-reduction techniques can mitigate the body's stress response and promote a sense of calm and relaxation. Here's how you can seamlessly integrate these elements into your lifestyle:

Exercise for Cortisol Regulation

1. Regular Aerobic Exercise:

Engage in moderate aerobic activities such as brisk walking, jogging, cycling, or swimming for at least 30 minutes on most days of the week. These exercises help increase heart rate and improve blood circulation, which can significantly lower stress levels and thus reduce cortisol over time.

2. Strength Training:

Incorporate strength training exercises two to three times per week. Building muscle helps improve metabolism and reduces fat, both of which can be adversely affected by high cortisol levels. Focus on major muscle groups and use free weights, resistance bands, or body-weight exercises like squats, push-ups, and lunges.

3. Yoga and Pilates:

Yoga and Pilates are excellent for stress reduction and flexibility. They combine physical postures with breathing techniques, improving physical strength and flexibility while also promoting relaxation and stress management.

4. Mindful Movement:

Activities like Tai Chi and Qigong focus on gentle movements, controlled breathing, and meditation. They are particularly effective at reducing stress, enhancing mental focus, and lowering cortisol.

Stress-Reducing Techniques

1. Deep Breathing Exercises:

Simple deep breathing techniques can be remarkably effective in managing acute stress. Techniques like diaphragmatic breathing (deep belly breathing) encourage full oxygen exchange and can slow the heartbeat and stabilize or even lower blood pressure, calming the stress response.

2. Progressive Muscle Relaxation (PMR):

This technique involves tensing and then relaxing different muscle groups in the body, which can help calm the mind and reduce overall bodily tension and stress.

3. Meditation and Mindfulness:

Regular meditation has been shown to reduce cortisol levels by improving relaxation and decreasing stress. Mindfulness meditation, in particular, focuses on being intensely aware of what you're sensing and feeling in the moment, without interpretation or judgment, and can be practiced anywhere at any time.

4. Guided Imagery:

This involves focusing your imagination on calm, peaceful settings or scenarios to help reduce feelings of stress. It's a powerful way to invoke positive, relaxing images that can help shift away from stressors.

5. Adequate Sleep:

Ensure you get enough sleep, as sleep deprivation can significantly increase cortisol levels. Aim for 7-9 hours per night, and try to keep a consistent sleep schedule, even on weekends.

6. Time in Nature:

Spending time outdoors, especially in green spaces, can reduce stress hormones and improve feelings of well-being. Even short periods spent in a park or garden can help.

7. Hobbies and Leisure Activities:

Engage regularly in activities you enjoy. Be it reading, painting, gardening, or playing music, hobbies can provide a great outlet for stress.

Integration Tips

To effectively integrate these practices, make them a part of your daily schedule. Even on busy days, a few minutes of breathing exercises or a short walk can make a big difference.

BREAKFAST IDEAS

Overnight Oats with Chia Seeds, Berries, and Almonds

Servings: 2

Prep Time: 10 minutes

Total Time: 8 hours 10 minutes (including overnight soaking)

Ingredients:

- 1 cup rolled oats
- 2 tablespoons chia seeds
- 1 cup mixed berries (fresh or frozen)
- 1/4 cup almonds, chopped
- 1 1/2 cups almond milk or milk of choice
- 1 tablespoon honey or maple syrup (optional)

Instructions:

1. In a large bowl or mason jar, combine rolled oats, chia seeds, mixed berries, and almonds.
2. Add almond milk and honey (if using), and stir to combine.

3. Cover and refrigerate overnight.

4. In the morning, stir the oats and add additional milk if needed for desired consistency.

5. Serve cold, topped with extra berries and almonds if desired.

Tips and Variations:

1. Substitute any type of nut or seed for the almonds if desired.

2. For a vegan version, ensure to use maple syrup instead of honey.

3. Add a scoop of protein powder for an extra protein boost.

Nutritional Information (per serving): Calories: 350 Protein: 10g, Fat: 15g, Saturated Fat: 1.5g, Cholesterol: 0mg, Carbohydrates: 45g, Fiber: 9g, Sugar: 12g, Sodium: 100mg

Spinach and Mushroom Omelet

Servings: 1

Prep Time: 5 minutes

Cook Time: 10 minutes

Total Time: 15 minutes

Ingredients:

- 2 large eggs
- 1/2 cup fresh spinach, chopped
- 1/4 cup mushrooms, sliced
- 1 tablespoon onion, chopped
- 1 tablespoon olive oil
- Salt and pepper, to taste
- 1 tablespoon grated cheese (optional)

Instructions:

1. In a medium skillet, heat olive oil over medium heat.
2. Add onions and mushrooms, and sauté until tender, about 5 minutes.
3. Add spinach and cook until wilted, about 2 minutes.

4. In a small bowl, beat the eggs with salt and pepper.

5. Pour the eggs over the vegetables in the skillet.

6. Cook until the eggs are set, about 3 minutes. Sprinkle with cheese if using.

7. Fold the omelet in half and serve hot.

Tips and Variations:

1. Add diced tomatoes or bell peppers for extra flavor and color.

2. For a dairy-free option, skip the cheese or use a dairy-free cheese alternative.

Nutritional Information (per serving): Calories: 280 Protein: 16g, Fat: 22g, Saturated Fat: 5g, Cholesterol: 370mg, Carbohydrates: 5g, Fiber: 1g, Sugar: 2g,Sodium: 320mg

Greek Yogurt with Flaxseeds and Honey

Servings: 1

Prep Time: 5 minutes

Total Time: 5 minutes

Ingredients:

- 1 cup Greek yogurt
- 1 tablespoon flaxseeds
- 2 teaspoons honey
- Optional toppings: fresh fruit, nuts, or granola

Instructions:

1. Place Greek yogurt in a serving bowl.
2. Sprinkle flaxseeds over the yogurt.
3. Drizzle honey on top.
4. Add optional toppings as desired.

Tips and Variations:

1. For added texture and flavor, include a handful of your favorite nuts or some granola.

2. Mix in some cinnamon or vanilla extract for a flavor boost.

Nutritional Information (per serving): Calories: 180
Protein: 20g, Fat: 4g, Saturated Fat: 1g, Cholesterol: 10mg
Carbohydrates: 18g, Fiber: 2g, Sugar: 15g
Sodium: 50mg

Avocado Toast on Whole Grain Bread with Poached Egg

Servings: 1

Prep Time: 5 minutes

Cook Time: 5 minutes

Total Time: 10 minutes

Ingredients:

- 1 slice whole grain bread
- 1/2 ripe avocado, mashed
- 1 egg
- Salt and pepper, to taste
- Optional: sprinkle of red pepper flakes or chopped herbs

Instructions:

1. Toast the whole grain bread to your preference.
2. While the bread is toasting, poach the egg in simmering water until the whites are set but the yolk remains runny, about 3-4 minutes.
3. Spread the mashed avocado on the toasted bread.
4. Top with the poached egg.

5. Season with salt, pepper, and optional red pepper flakes or herbs.

Tips and Variations:
1. Add sliced tomatoes or radishes for extra freshness and crunch.
2. For extra protein, add a slice of smoked salmon beneath the egg.

Nutritional Information (per serving): Calories: 300, Protein: 13g, Fat: 20g, Saturated Fat: 3.5g, Cholesterol: 185mg, Carbohydrates: 22g, Fiber: 7g, Sugar: 3g, Sodium: 400mg

Quinoa Porridge with Apples and Cinnamon

Servings: 2

Prep Time: 5 minutes

Cook Time: 15 minutes

Total Time: 20 minutes

Ingredients:

- 1 cup quinoa, rinsed
- 2 cups almond milk
- 1 apple, peeled, cored, and diced
- 1/2 teaspoon cinnamon
- 1 tablespoon honey or maple syrup
- Optional: a pinch of nutmeg

Instructions:

1. In a medium saucepan, combine quinoa and almond milk. Bring to a boil over high heat.
2. Reduce heat to low, cover, and simmer for 15 minutes, or until most of the liquid is absorbed.
3. Stir in diced apple, cinnamon, and honey or maple syrup. Cook for an additional 5 minutes.

4. Serve hot, with an optional pinch of nutmeg sprinkled on top.

Tips and Variations:
1. Mix in a tablespoon of chia seeds for extra fiber.
2. Top with chopped nuts or a dollop of yogurt for added texture and flavor.

Nutritional Information (per serving): Calories: 285
Protein: 8g, Fat: 5g, Saturated Fat: 0g, Cholesterol: 0mg
Carbohydrates: 53g, Fiber: 6g, Sugar: 15g, Sodium: 150mg

Greek Yogurt with Flaxseeds and Honey

Servings: 1

Prep Time: 5 minutes

Total Time: 5 minutes

Ingredients:

- 1 cup Greek yogurt
- 1 tablespoon flaxseeds
- 2 teaspoons honey
- Optional toppings: fresh fruit, nuts, or granola

Instructions:

1. Place Greek yogurt in a serving bowl.
2. Sprinkle flaxseeds over the yogurt.
3. Drizzle honey on top.
4. Add optional toppings as desired.

Tips and Variations:

1. For added texture and flavor, include a handful of your favorite nuts or some granola.

2. Mix in some cinnamon or vanilla extract for a flavor boost.

Nutritional Information (per serving): Calories: 180
Protein: 20g, Fat: 4g, Saturated Fat: 1g, Cholesterol: 10mg
Carbohydrates: 18g, Fiber: 2g, Sugar: 15g, Sodium: 50mg

Avocado Toast on Whole Grain Bread with Poached Egg

Servings: 1

Prep Time: 5 minutes

Cook Time: 5 minutes

Total Time: 10 minutes

Ingredients:

- 1 slice whole grain bread
- 1/2 ripe avocado, mashed
- 1 egg
- Salt and pepper, to taste
- Optional: sprinkle of red pepper flakes or chopped herbs

Instructions:

1. Toast the whole grain bread to your preference.
2. While the bread is toasting, poach the egg in simmering water until the whites are set but the yolk remains runny, about 3-4 minutes.
3. Spread the mashed avocado on the toasted bread.
4. Top with the poached egg.

5. Season with salt, pepper, and optional red pepper flakes or herbs.

Tips and Variations:
1. Add sliced tomatoes or radishes for extra freshness and crunch.
2. For extra protein, add a slice of smoked salmon beneath the egg.

Nutritional Information (per serving): Calories: 300 Protein: 13g, Fat: 20g, Saturated Fat: 3.5g, Cholesterol: 185mg, Carbohydrates: 22g, Fiber: 7g, Sugar: 3g, Sodium: 400mg

Quinoa Porridge with Apples and Cinnamon

Servings: 2

Prep Time: 5 minutes

Cook Time: 15 minutes

Total Time: 20 minutes

Ingredients:

- 1 cup quinoa, rinsed
- 2 cups almond milk
- 1 apple, peeled, cored, and diced
- 1/2 teaspoon cinnamon
- 1 tablespoon honey or maple syrup
- Optional: a pinch of nutmeg

Instructions:

1. In a medium saucepan, combine quinoa and almond milk. Bring to a boil over high heat.
2. Reduce heat to low, cover, and simmer for 15 minutes, or until most of the liquid is absorbed.
3. Stir in diced apple, cinnamon, and honey or maple syrup. Cook for an additional 5 minutes.

4. Serve hot, with an optional pinch of nutmeg sprinkled on top.

Tips and Variations:
1. Mix in a tablespoon of chia seeds for extra fiber.
2. Top with chopped nuts or a dollop of yogurt for added texture and flavor.

Nutritional Information (per serving): Calories: 285
Protein: 8g, Fat: 5g, Saturated Fat: 0g, Cholesterol: 0mg
Carbohydrates: 53g, Fiber: 6g, Sugar: 15g, Sodium: 150mg

Smoothie Bowl with Kale, Banana, and Peanut Butter

Servings: 1

Prep Time: 10 minutes

Total Time: 10 minutes

Ingredients:

- 1 cup kale, stems removed
- 1 ripe banana
- 1 tablespoon peanut butter
- 1/2 cup almond milk or milk of choice
- 1/2 cup ice
- Optional toppings: sliced banana, granola, chia seeds

Instructions:

1. In a blender, combine kale, banana, peanut butter, almond milk, and ice.
2. Blend on high until smooth and creamy.
3. Pour the smoothie into a bowl.
4. Top with optional toppings such as sliced banana, granola, and chia seeds as desired.

Tips and Variations:

1. For a protein boost, add a scoop of your favorite protein powder.

2. Substitute spinach for kale if preferred, or use a mix of both for varied nutrients.

Nutritional Information (per serving): Calories: 280
Protein: 8g, Fat: 10g, Saturated Fat: 2g, Cholesterol: 0mg
Carbohydrates: 44g, Fiber: 7g, Sugar: 21g, Sodium: 150mg

Whole Grain Pancakes with Fresh Berries

Servings: 4

Prep Time: 10 minutes

Cook Time: 15 minutes

Total Time: 25 minutes

Ingredients:

- 1 cup whole grain flour
- 1 teaspoon baking powder
- 1/2 teaspoon baking soda
- 1/4 teaspoon salt
- 1 tablespoon sugar (optional)
- 1 large egg, beaten
- 1 cup buttermilk
- 2 tablespoons unsalted butter, melted
- 1 cup mixed fresh berries (such as blueberries, strawberries, and raspberries)
- Maple syrup, for serving

Instructions:

1. In a large bowl, whisk together the flour, baking powder, baking soda, salt, and sugar if using.

2. In another bowl, combine the beaten egg, buttermilk, and melted butter.

3. Add the wet ingredients to the dry ingredients and stir until just combined.

4. Heat a non-stick skillet or griddle over medium heat. Pour 1/4 cup of batter for each pancake.

5. Cook until bubbles form on the surface, then flip and cook until golden brown on the other side.

6. Serve hot with fresh berries and maple syrup.

Tips and Variations:

1. Add a dash of cinnamon or vanilla extract to the batter for extra flavor.

2. For a dairy-free version, use almond milk and a plant-based butter alternative.

Nutritional Information (per serving): Calories: 250
Protein: 8g, Fat: 9g, Saturated Fat: 5g, Cholesterol: 60mg
Carbohydrates: 35g, Fiber: 5g, Sugar: 10g, Sodium: 400mg

Baked Sweet Potato Hash with Eggs

Servings: 2

Prep Time: 10 minutes

Cook Time: 25 minutes

Total Time: 35 minutes

Ingredients:

- 2 medium sweet potatoes, peeled and diced
- 1 small onion, diced
- 1 red bell pepper, diced
- 2 tablespoons olive oil
- Salt and pepper, to taste
- 4 eggs
- Optional: chopped fresh herbs such as parsley or chives

Instructions:

1. Preheat the oven to 400°F (200°C).
2. On a baking sheet, toss the sweet potatoes, onion, and bell pepper with olive oil, salt, and pepper.

3. Roast in the preheated oven for 20 minutes, or until the vegetables are tender and starting to brown.
4. Remove from the oven and make four wells in the hash. Crack an egg into each well.
5. Return to the oven and bake for an additional 5-7 minutes, or until the egg whites are set but yolks are still runny.
6. Serve hot, garnished with optional fresh herbs.

Tips and Variations:
1. Add diced chorizo or bacon to the hash for extra flavor.
2. For a spicy kick, sprinkle some crushed red pepper flakes before baking.

Nutritional Information (per serving): Calories: 320 Protein: 15g, Fat: 18g, Saturated Fat: 4g, Cholesterol: 370mg, Carbohydrates: 27g, Fiber: 4g, Sugar: 8g, Sodium: 200mg

Turkey Sausage and Bell Peppers Scramble

Servings: 2

Prep Time: 5 minutes

Cook Time: 10 minutes

Total Time: 15 minutes

Ingredients:

- 4 turkey sausages, casings removed
- 1 red bell pepper, diced
- 1 green bell pepper, diced
- 4 large eggs
- 1 tablespoon olive oil
- Salt and pepper, to taste

Instructions:

1. Heat olive oil in a skillet over medium heat.
2. Add the turkey sausages and break them up with a spoon. Cook until browned and cooked through.
3. Add the diced bell peppers to the skillet and sauté until they are soft.

4. Beat the eggs in a bowl and pour over the sausage and peppers in the skillet.
5. Stir gently until the eggs are fully cooked.
6. Season with salt and pepper to taste and serve immediately.

Tips and Variations:
1. Add onions or mushrooms for extra flavor and texture.
2. Top with shredded cheese or fresh herbs like chives or parsley before serving.

Nutritional Information (per serving): Calories: 400 Protein: 35g, Fat: 25g, Saturated Fat: 7g, Cholesterol: 430mg, Carbohydrates: 8g, Fiber: 2g, Sugar: 4g, Sodium: 870mg

Pumpkin Spice Oatmeal

Servings: 2

Prep Time: 5 minutes

Cook Time: 10 minutes

Total Time: 15 minutes

Ingredients:

- 1 cup rolled oats
- 1 3/4 cups milk or water
- 1/2 cup pure pumpkin puree
- 1 teaspoon pumpkin pie spice
- 1 tablespoon maple syrup
- Optional toppings: chopped nuts, dried cranberries, a dollop of yogurt

Instructions:

1. In a medium saucepan, bring milk or water to a boil.
2. Add rolled oats and reduce heat to a simmer.
3. Stir in pumpkin puree and pumpkin pie spice.
4. Cook for about 5-7 minutes until the oats are soft and the mixture has thickened.

5. Remove from heat and stir in maple syrup.

6. Serve hot, garnished with optional toppings as desired.

Tips and Variations:

1. Substitute almond milk for a dairy-free version.

2. Add a scoop of protein powder for an extra protein boost.

3. Sweeten with honey or agave syrup instead of maple syrup if preferred.

Nutritional Information (per serving): Calories: 280
Protein: 10g, Fat: 5g, Saturated Fat: 2g, Cholesterol: 10mg
Carbohydrates: 50g, Fiber: 6g, Sugar: 12g, Sodium: 70mg

Whole Grain Waffles with Ricotta and Strawberries

Servings: 4

Prep Time: 10 minutes

Cook Time: 15 minutes

Total Time: 25 minutes

Ingredients:

- 1 1/2 cups whole grain flour
- 2 teaspoons baking powder
- 1/2 teaspoon salt
- 2 tablespoons sugar
- 1 large egg
- 1 cup milk
- 1/4 cup vegetable oil
- 1/2 cup ricotta cheese
- 1 cup sliced strawberries

Instructions:

1. In a large bowl, whisk together flour, baking powder, salt, and sugar.

2. In another bowl, beat the egg with milk and vegetable oil.

3. Add the wet ingredients to the dry ingredients, mixing until just combined.

4. Preheat a waffle iron and grease it lightly.

5. Pour enough batter to cover the waffle iron surface, close the lid, and cook until the waffle is golden and crisp.

6. Serve waffles topped with ricotta cheese and sliced strawberries.

Tips and Variations:

1. Add vanilla extract or cinnamon to the batter for additional flavor.

2. Top with blueberries or bananas instead of strawberries for variety.

Nutritional Information (per serving): Calories: 390
Protein: 12g, Fat: 20g, Saturated Fat: 5g, Cholesterol: 60mg
Carbohydrates: 44g, Fiber: 6g, Sugar: 10g, Sodium: 350mg

Tofu and Vegetable Stir-fry with Tamari Sauce

Servings: 2

Prep Time: 10 minutes

Cook Time: 10 minutes

Total Time: 20 minutes

Ingredients:

- 1 block firm tofu, drained and cubed
- 1 tablespoon vegetable oil
- 1 bell pepper, sliced
- 1 zucchini, sliced
- 1 carrot, julienned
- 2 tablespoons tamari or soy sauce
- 1 teaspoon sesame oil
- 1 clove garlic, minced
- 1 teaspoon fresh ginger, grated
- Optional: sesame seeds, green onions for garnish

Instructions:

1. Heat vegetable oil in a large skillet over medium-high heat.

2. Add tofu cubes and cook until golden brown on all sides, about 5 minutes.

3. Add bell pepper, zucchini, and carrot to the skillet. Stir-fry for about 5 minutes, until vegetables are tender-crisp.

4. Lower the heat to medium. Add tamari, sesame oil, garlic, and ginger. Stir well to combine and coat the tofu and vegetables.

5. Cook for an additional 2 minutes, then remove from heat.

6. Serve hot, garnished with sesame seeds and green onions if desired.

Tips and Variations:

1. Include broccoli or snap peas for extra crunch and nutrition.

2. For a spicier version, add a splash of chili sauce or a pinch of red pepper flakes.

Nutritional Information (per serving): Calories: 300
Protein: 18g, Fat: 18g, Saturated Fat: 2g, Cholesterol: 0mg
Carbohydrates: 20g, Fiber: 4g, Sugar: 6g, Sodium: 870mg

Protein Smoothie with Spinach, Blueberry, and Yogurt

Servings: 1

Prep Time: 5 minutes

Total Time: 5 minutes

Ingredients:

- 1 cup fresh spinach
- 1/2 cup blueberries
- 1 banana
- 1/2 cup Greek yogurt
- 1/2 cup water or almond milk
- 1 scoop protein powder (optional)

Instructions:

1. Place all ingredients in a blender.
2. Blend on high until smooth.
3. Serve immediately.

Tips and Variations:

1. Add a tablespoon of flaxseeds or chia seeds for extra fiber and omega-3 fatty acids.
2. Replace blueberries with any other berries of your choice for different flavors.

Nutritional Information (per serving): Calories: 290 Protein: 20g (if using protein powder), Fat: 2g Saturated Fat: 0g, Cholesterol: 5mg, Carbohydrates: 46g, Fiber: 7g, Sugar: 28g, Sodium: 70mg

LUNCH AND DINNER RECIPES

Grilled Chicken Salad with Mixed Greens and Avocado

Servings: 4

Prep Time: 15 minutes

Cook Time: 10 minutes

Total Time: 25 minutes

Ingredients:

- 1-pound boneless, skinless chicken breasts
- 1 tablespoon olive oil
- Salt and pepper, to taste
- 4 cups mixed greens (such as arugula, spinach, and romaine)
- 1 ripe avocado, sliced
- 1/2 red onion, thinly sliced
- 1/2 cup cherry tomatoes, halved
- 1/4 cup balsamic vinaigrette

Instructions:

1. Preheat grill to medium-high heat.
2. Brush chicken breasts with olive oil and season with salt and pepper.
3. Grill chicken for 5 minutes on each side or until fully cooked and juices run clear.
4. Let chicken rest for 5 minutes, then slice.
5. In a large bowl, toss mixed greens, avocado slices, red onion, and cherry tomatoes.
6. Top salad with sliced grilled chicken.
7. Drizzle with balsamic vinaigrette and serve.

Tips and Variations:

1. Add crumbled goat cheese or feta for extra flavor.
2. Include nuts such as walnuts or almonds for added crunch.

Nutritional Information (per serving): Calories: 290
Protein: 25g, Fat: 15g, Saturated Fat: 2g, Cholesterol: 65mg
Carbohydrates: 12g, Fiber: 4g, Sugar: 5g, Sodium: 220mg

Quinoa and Black Bean Wrap with Salsa

Servings: 4

Prep Time: 15 minutes

Cook Time: 0 minutes

Total Time: 15 minutes

Ingredients:

- 2 cups cooked quinoa
- 1 can (15 oz) black beans, rinsed and drained
- 1 avocado, diced
- 1/2 cup corn kernels
- 1/2 cup fresh salsa
- 4 whole wheat wraps
- 1/4 cup chopped cilantro
- Juice of 1 lime
- Salt and pepper, to taste

Instructions:

1. In a large bowl, mix quinoa, black beans, avocado, corn, salsa, cilantro, and lime juice. Season with salt and pepper.

2. Spoon the mixture evenly onto the center of each wrap.

3. Fold the bottom edge of the wrap tightly over the filling, then fold in the sides and roll up securely.

4. Serve immediately or wrap in foil to take on the go.

Tips and Variations:

1. Add a dollop of Greek yogurt or sour cream for creaminess.

2. Spice it up with jalapeños or a dash of hot sauce.

Nutritional Information (per serving): Calories: 360 Protein: 12g, Fat: 10g, Saturated Fat: 1.5g, Cholesterol: 0mg, Carbohydrates: 56g, Fiber: 10g, Sugar: 3g, Sodium: 420mg

Broccoli and Almond Soup

Servings: 4

Prep Time: 10 minutes

Cook Time: 20 minutes

Total Time: 30 minutes

Ingredients:

- 2 tablespoons olive oil
- 1 onion, chopped
- 2 cloves garlic, minced
- 4 cups broccoli florets
- 4 cups vegetable broth
- 1/2 cup almonds, toasted and chopped
- Salt and pepper, to taste
- Optional: 1/4 cup heavy cream for garnish

Instructions:

1. In a large pot, heat olive oil over medium heat. Add onion and garlic, sauté until onion is translucent.

2. Add broccoli and vegetable broth. Bring to a boil, then reduce heat and simmer until broccoli is tender, about 15 minutes.
3. Use an immersion blender to puree the soup until smooth.
4. Stir in chopped almonds, and season with salt and pepper to taste.
5. Serve hot, with a drizzle of heavy cream if desired.

Tips and Variations:
1. For a nuttier flavor, add more almonds or even a spoonful of almond butter.
2. If you prefer a thinner soup, adjust the consistency with additional vegetable broth.

Nutritional Information (per serving): Calories: 230 Protein: 8g, Fat: 18g, Saturated Fat: 3g, Cholesterol: 10mg Carbohydrates: 14g, Fiber: 5g, Sugar: 4g, Sodium: 400mg

Turkey and Hummus Sandwich on Whole Grain Bread

Servings: 2

Prep Time: 5 minutes

Cook Time: 0 minutes

Total Time: 5 minutes

Ingredients:

- 4 slices whole grain bread
- 4 tablespoons hummus
- 4 slices turkey breast
- 1 tomato, sliced
- 1/2 cucumber, sliced
- 1/4 red onion, thinly sliced
- Salt and pepper, to taste

Instructions:

1. Spread hummus evenly on each slice of whole grain bread.
2. Layer turkey slices, tomato slices, cucumber slices, and red onion on two slices of bread.
3. Season with salt and pepper.

4. Top with the remaining slices of bread, hummus side down.

5. Cut sandwiches in half and serve.

Tips and Variations:

1. Add lettuce, spinach, or arugula for additional greens.

2. Try different flavors of hummus, such as roasted red pepper or garlic, for variety.

Nutritional Information (per serving): Calories: 350 Protein: 25g, Fat: 9g, Saturated Fat: 1.5g, Cholesterol: 35mg, Carbohydrates: 42g, Fiber: 8g, Sugar: 8g, Sodium: 890mg

Lentil and Vegetable Stew

Servings: 4

Prep Time: 15 minutes

Cook Time: 45 minutes

Total Time: 1 hour

Ingredients:

- 1 tablespoon olive oil
- 1 onion, chopped
- 2 carrots, diced
- 2 celery stalks, diced
- 2 cloves garlic, minced
- 1 teaspoon dried thyme
- 1 cup dried lentils, rinsed
- 4 cups vegetable broth
- 1 can (14.5 oz) diced tomatoes
- Salt and pepper, to taste
- Optional: chopped fresh parsley for garnish

Instructions:

1. In a large pot, heat olive oil over medium heat. Add onion, carrots, celery, and garlic; sauté until vegetables are softened, about 5 minutes.
2. Stir in thyme and lentils, then add vegetable broth and diced tomatoes. Bring to a boil.
3. Reduce heat, cover, and simmer until lentils are tender, about 35 minutes.
4. Season with salt and pepper to taste.
5. Serve hot, garnished with fresh parsley if desired.

Tips and Variations:

1. Add spinach or kale during the last 10 minutes of cooking for added greens.
2. For a non-vegetarian version, add diced cooked chicken or turkey.

Nutritional Information (per serving): Calories: 250 Protein: 15g, Fat: 4g, Saturated Fat: 0.5g, Cholesterol: 0mg Carbohydrates: 40g, Fiber: 15g, Sugar: 8g, Sodium: 700mg

Grilled Salmon with Asparagus and Quinoa

Servings: 4

Prep Time: 10 minutes

Cook Time: 20 minutes

Total Time: 30 minutes

Ingredients:

- 4 salmon fillets (about 6 ounces each)
- 1 tablespoon olive oil
- Salt and pepper, to taste
- 1 pound asparagus, trimmed
- 2 cups cooked quinoa
- Lemon wedges, for serving

Instructions:

1. Preheat grill to medium-high heat.
2. Brush salmon fillets and asparagus with olive oil and season with salt and pepper.
3. Grill salmon, skin side down, for 6-8 minutes. Flip and cook for an additional 4-6 minutes, or until salmon is opaque and flakes easily with a fork.

4. Grill asparagus alongside salmon for about 5-7 minutes, turning occasionally, until tender and charred.

5. Serve grilled salmon and asparagus over a bed of quinoa, with lemon wedges on the side.

Tips and Variations:

1. Drizzle a mixture of Dijon mustard and honey over the salmon before grilling for added flavor.

2. Mix fresh herbs such as parsley or dill into the quinoa for extra freshness.

Nutritional Information (per serving): Calories: 450 Protein: 38g, Fat: 20g, Saturated Fat: 3g, Cholesterol: 85mg Carbohydrates: 30g, Fiber: 5g, Sugar: 3g, Sodium: 75mg

Baked Cod with Lemon and Dill, served with Steamed Broccoli

Servings: 4

Prep Time: 10 minutes

Cook Time: 20 minutes

Total Time: 30 minutes

Ingredients:

- 4 cod fillets (about 6 ounces each)
- 2 tablespoons olive oil
- Juice and zest of 1 lemon
- 2 tablespoons fresh dill, chopped
- Salt and pepper, to taste
- 4 cups broccoli florets

Instructions:

1. Preheat oven to 400°F (200°C).
2. Place cod fillets in a baking dish. Drizzle with olive oil and lemon juice, and sprinkle with lemon zest, dill, salt, and pepper.
3. Bake in preheated oven for 12-15 minutes, or until cod is opaque and flakes easily with a fork.

4. While cod is baking, steam broccoli until tender, about 5-7 minutes.

5. Serve baked cod with steamed broccoli on the side.

Tips and Variations:
1. Add capers or sliced olives to the baking dish before cooking for a Mediterranean twist.

2. Substitute parsley or chives for dill if preferred.

Nutritional Information (per serving): Calories: 250 Protein: 28g, Fat: 10g, Saturated Fat: 1.5g, Cholesterol: 60mg, Carbohydrates: 10g, Fiber: 3g, Sugar: 2g, Sodium: 200mg

Stuffed Bell Peppers with Ground Chicken and Vegetables

Servings: 4

Prep Time: 15 minutes

Cook Time: 30 minutes

Total Time: 45 minutes

Ingredients:

- 4 bell peppers, tops cut off and seeds removed
- 1 pound ground chicken
- 1 tablespoon olive oil
- 1 onion, finely chopped
- 2 cloves garlic, minced
- 1 cup cooked rice
- 1 zucchini, diced
- 1 cup tomato sauce
- 1 teaspoon dried basil
- Salt and pepper, to taste
- 1/2 cup shredded mozzarella cheese (optional)

Instructions:

1. Preheat oven to 375°F (190°C).

2. In a skillet, heat olive oil over medium heat. Add onion and garlic, and sauté until translucent.

3. Add ground chicken and cook until browned.

4. Stir in cooked rice, zucchini, tomato sauce, basil, salt, and pepper. Cook until mixture is heated through.

5. Spoon the filling into each bell pepper and place in a baking dish.

6. Top with shredded mozzarella cheese if using.

7. Cover with foil and bake for 25 minutes. Remove foil and bake for an additional 5 minutes or until cheese is bubbly and golden. Serve hot.

Tips and Variations:

1. Substitute ground turkey or beef for chicken if desired.

2. Add other vegetables like corn or carrots to the filling for more variety and nutrition.

Nutritional Information (per serving): Calories: 360 Protein: 26g, Fat: 18g, Saturated Fat: 5g Cholesterol: 80mg, Carbohydrates: 22g, Fiber: 4g, Sugar: 8g, Sodium: 400mg

Grilled Shrimp and Vegetable Kabobs

Servings: 4

Prep Time: 20 minutes (plus marinating time)

Cook Time: 10 minutes

Total Time: 30 minutes

Ingredients:

-   1 pound shrimp, peeled and deveined
-   1 zucchini, cut into 1-inch slices
-   1 red bell pepper, cut into 1-inch pieces
-   1 yellow bell pepper, cut into 1-inch pieces
-   1 onion, cut into 1-inch pieces
-   1/4 cup olive oil
-   2 tablespoons lemon juice
-   2 cloves garlic, minced
-   1 teaspoon dried oregano
-   Salt and pepper, to taste

Instructions:

1. In a bowl, whisk together olive oil, lemon juice, garlic, oregano, salt, and pepper.

2. Add shrimp and vegetables to the marinade and toss to coat. Let marinate for at least 30 minutes.
3. Preheat grill to medium-high heat.
4. Thread shrimp and vegetables alternately onto skewers.
5. Grill kabobs, turning occasionally, until shrimp is cooked through and vegetables are tender, about 10 minutes.
6. Serve hot.

Tips and Variations:
1. Use metal skewers or soak wooden skewers in water for 30 minutes before threading to prevent burning.
2. Serve with a side of rice or a fresh salad for a complete meal.

Nutritional Information (per serving): Calories: 290
Protein: 24g, Fat: 18g, Saturated Fat: 3g, Cholesterol: 145mg, Carbohydrates: 10g, Fiber: 2g, Sugar: 4g, Sodium: 880mg

Vegetarian Chili with Avocado and Cornbread

Servings: 4

Prep Time: 15 minutes

Cook Time: 35 minutes

Total Time: 50 minutes

Ingredients:

- 1 tablespoon olive oil
- 1 onion, chopped
- 2 cloves garlic, minced
- 1 bell pepper, chopped
- 1 zucchini, chopped
- 2 carrots, chopped
- 1 can (15 oz) black beans, drained and rinsed
- 1 can (15 oz) kidney beans, drained and rinsed
- 1 can (28 oz) crushed tomatoes
- 2 tablespoons chili powder
- 1 teaspoon cumin
- Salt and pepper, to taste
- 1 ripe avocado, diced
- Cornbread, for serving

Instructions:

1. Heat olive oil in a large pot over medium heat.
2. Add onion, garlic, bell pepper, zucchini, and carrots. Sauté until vegetables are softened, about 5 minutes.
3. Add black beans, kidney beans, crushed tomatoes, chili powder, and cumin. Stir to combine.
4. Bring to a boil, then reduce heat and simmer for 30 minutes, stirring occasionally.
5. Season with salt and pepper to taste.
6. Serve hot, topped with diced avocado and a side of cornbread.

Tips and Variations:

1. Add a can of corn or other vegetables for more texture and flavor.
2. Top with shredded cheese or a dollop of sour cream for extra richness.

Nutritional Information (per serving): Calories: 380 Protein: 15g, Fat: 15g, Saturated Fat: 2g, Cholesterol: 0mg Carbohydrates: 52g, Fiber: 15g, Sugar: 12g, Sodium: 780mg

Roasted Chicken with Sweet Potatoes and Brussels Sprouts

Servings: 4

Prep Time: 10 minutes

Cook Time: 45 minutes

Total Time: 55 minutes

Ingredients:

- 4 chicken thighs, bone-in and skin-on
- 2 sweet potatoes, peeled and cubed
- 2 cups Brussels sprouts, halved
- 2 tablespoons olive oil
- 1 teaspoon garlic powder
- 1 teaspoon dried rosemary
- Salt and pepper, to taste

Instructions:

1. Preheat oven to 400°F (200°C).
2. Arrange chicken thighs, sweet potatoes, and Brussels sprouts on a large baking sheet.

3. Drizzle with olive oil and sprinkle with garlic powder, rosemary, salt, and pepper. Toss to coat evenly.
4. Roast in the preheated oven for 45 minutes, or until the chicken is golden and cooked through and vegetables are tender and caramelized.
5. Serve hot.

Tips and Variations:
1. Swap sweet potatoes for butternut squash or carrots for a different flavor profile.
2. Add a splash of balsamic vinegar in the last 10 minutes of roasting for a touch of acidity.

Nutritional Information (per serving): Calories: 450 Protein: 25g, Fat: 25g, Saturated Fat: 6g, Cholesterol: 140mg, Carbohydrates: 33g, Fiber: 6g, Sugar: 7g, Sodium: 300mg

Beef Stir-fry with Bell Peppers and Brown Rice

Servings: 4

Prep Time: 15 minutes

Cook Time: 20 minutes

Total Time: 35 minutes

Ingredients:

- 1 pound beef sirloin, thinly sliced
- 2 tablespoons vegetable oil
- 1 red bell pepper, sliced
- 1 green bell pepper, sliced
- 1 onion, sliced
- 2 cloves garlic, minced
- 2 tablespoons soy sauce
- 1 tablespoon oyster sauce
- 1 teaspoon sesame oil
- 1 cup brown rice, cooked according to package instructions

Instructions:

1. Heat 1 tablespoon of vegetable oil in a large skillet or wok over high heat.

2. Add beef slices and stir-fry until browned and cooked through, about 3-4 minutes. Remove beef from the skillet and set aside.

3. In the same skillet, add the remaining tablespoon of vegetable oil. Add red and green bell peppers, onion, and garlic. Stir-fry until vegetables are tender but still crisp, about 5-7 minutes.

4. Return the beef to the skillet. Add soy sauce, oyster sauce, and sesame oil. Stir well to combine and heat through.

5. Serve the beef stir-fry over cooked brown rice.

Tips and Variations:

Add a splash of chili sauce or a pinch of red pepper flakes to add some heat to the dish.

Include other vegetables like broccoli, snap peas, or carrots for added nutrition and color.

Nutritional Information (per serving): Calories: 380 Protein: 26g, Fat: 15g, Saturated Fat: 3g, Cholesterol: 70mg, Carbohydrates: 35g, Fiber: 4g, Sugar: 3g, Sodium: 650mg

Pork Tenderloin with Apple Sauce and Roasted Carrots

Servings: 4

Prep Time: 10 minutes

Cook Time: 25 minutes

Total Time: 35 minutes

Ingredients:

- 1 pork tenderloin (about 1 pound)
- 2 tablespoons olive oil
- Salt and pepper, to taste
- 4 carrots, peeled and sliced
- 1 cup apple sauce

Instructions:

1. Preheat oven to 375°F (190°C).
2. Rub pork tenderloin with 1 tablespoon of olive oil, salt, and pepper. Place in a roasting pan.
3. Toss sliced carrots with the remaining tablespoon of olive oil, and arrange around the pork in the roasting pan.

4. Roast in the preheated oven for 25 minutes, or until the pork reaches an internal temperature of 145°F (63°C) and the carrots are tender.
5. Let the pork rest for 5 minutes before slicing.
6. Serve the pork slices with apple sauce and roasted carrots on the side.

Tips and Variations:
1. For added flavor, marinate the pork tenderloin in a mixture of apple cider vinegar, garlic, and herbs before roasting.
2. Substitute sweet potatoes or parsnips for the carrots, or include both for a hearty side.

Nutritional Information (per serving): Calories: 290
Protein: 24g, Fat: 13g, Saturated Fat: 3g, Cholesterol: 75mg
Carbohydrates: 19g, Fiber: 3g, Sugar: 12g, Sodium: 200mg

Butternut Squash Risotto

Servings: 4

Prep Time: 10 minutes

Cook Time: 30 minutes

Total Time: 40 minutes

Ingredients:

- 1 butternut squash, peeled and cubed (about 4 cups)
- 2 tablespoons olive oil, divided
- 1 small onion, finely chopped
- 1 cup Arborio rice
- 1/2 cup white wine
- 4 cups vegetable broth, kept warm
- 1/2 cup grated Parmesan cheese
- Salt and pepper, to taste
- Fresh sage, chopped, for garnish

Instructions:

1. Preheat oven to 400°F (200°C).
2. Toss butternut squash with 1 tablespoon of olive oil and season with salt and pepper. Spread on a baking sheet and roast until tender and lightly caramelized, about 20-25 minutes.

3. In a large saucepan, heat the remaining tablespoon of olive oil over medium heat. Add onion and sauté until translucent, about 5 minutes.

4. Add Arborio rice and stir to coat with the oil. Cook for 1-2 minutes until slightly toasted.

5. Add white wine and stir until mostly absorbed.

6. Add warm vegetable broth, one ladle at a time, stirring frequently. Wait until each addition is almost fully absorbed before adding the next.

7. When the rice is creamy and just tender (about 18-20 minutes), stir in the roasted butternut squash and Parmesan cheese. Adjust seasoning with salt and pepper. Serve hot, garnished with fresh sage.

Tips and Variations:

1. Add a handful of chopped spinach or kale in the last few minutes of cooking for extra greens.

2. Swap butternut squash for pumpkin or sweet potatoes for a different flavor profile.

Nutritional Information (per serving): Calories: 350
Protein: 9g, Fat: 12g, Saturated Fat: 3g, Cholesterol: 10mg
Carbohydrates: 53g, Fiber: 4g, Sugar: 5g, Sodium: 780mg

Grilled Shrimp and Vegetable Kabobs

Servings: 4

Prep Time: 20 minutes (plus marinating time)

Cook Time: 10 minutes

Total Time: 30 minutes

Ingredients:

- 1 pound shrimp, peeled and deveined
- 1 zucchini, cut into 1-inch slices
- 1 red bell pepper, cut into 1-inch pieces
- 1 yellow bell pepper, cut into 1-inch pieces
- 1 onion, cut into 1-inch pieces
- 1/4 cup olive oil
- 2 tablespoons lemon juice
- 2 cloves garlic, minced
- 1 teaspoon dried oregano
- Salt and pepper, to taste

Instructions:

1. In a bowl, whisk together olive oil, lemon juice, garlic, oregano, salt, and pepper.

2. Add shrimp and vegetables to the marinade and toss to coat. Let marinate for at least 30 minutes.
3. Preheat grill to medium-high heat.
4. Thread shrimp and vegetables alternately onto skewers.
5. Grill kabobs, turning occasionally, until shrimp is cooked through and vegetables are tender, about 10 minutes. Serve hot.

Tips and Variations:
1. Use metal skewers or soak wooden skewers in water for 30 minutes before threading to prevent burning.
2. Serve with a side of rice or a fresh salad for a complete meal.

Nutritional Information (per serving): Calories: 290 Protein: 24g, Fat: 18g, Saturated Fat: 3g, Cholesterol: 145mg, Carbohydrates: 10g, Fiber: 2g, Sugar: 4g Sodium: 880mg

Vegetarian Chili with Avocado and Cornbread

Servings: 4

Prep Time: 15 minutes

Cook Time: 35 minutes

Total Time: 50 minutes

Ingredients:

- 1 tablespoon olive oil
- 1 onion, chopped
- 2 cloves garlic, minced
- 1 bell pepper, chopped
- 1 zucchini, chopped
- 2 carrots, chopped
- 1 can (15 oz) black beans, drained and rinsed
- 1 can (15 oz) kidney beans, drained and rinsed
- 1 can (28 oz) crushed tomatoes
- 2 tablespoons chili powder
- 1 teaspoon cumin
- Salt and pepper, to taste
- 1 ripe avocado, diced
- Cornbread, for serving

Instructions:

1. Heat olive oil in a large pot over medium heat.
2. Add onion, garlic, bell pepper, zucchini, and carrots. Sauté until vegetables are softened, about 5 minutes.
3. Add black beans, kidney beans, crushed tomatoes, chili powder, and cumin. Stir to combine.
4. Bring to a boil, then reduce heat and simmer for 30 minutes, stirring occasionally.
5. Season with salt and pepper to taste.
6. Serve hot, topped with diced avocado and a side of cornbread.

Tips and Variations:

1. Add a can of corn or other vegetables for more texture and flavor.
2. Top with shredded cheese or a dollop of sour cream for extra richness.

Nutritional Information (per serving): Calories: 380
Protein: 15g, Fat: 15g, Saturated Fat: 2g, Cholesterol: 0mg
Carbohydrates: 52g, Fiber: 15g, Sugar: 12g, Sodium: 780mg

TASTY SNACK RECIPES

Almonds and Walnuts Mix

Servings: 4

Prep Time: 5 minutes

Total Time: 5 minutes

Ingredients:

- 1/2 cup raw almonds
- 1/2 cup raw walnuts

Instructions:

1. Combine almonds and walnuts in a bowl and mix well.
2. Divide into serving portions or store in an airtight container for a quick snack.

Tips and Variations:

1. Roast the nuts in the oven at 350°F for 10-12 minutes for added crunch and flavor.

Nutritional Information (per serving): Calories: 200
Protein: 6g, Fat: 18g, Saturated Fat: 2g, Carbohydrates: 6g,
Fiber: 3g, Sugar: 1g

Greek Yogurt with Mixed Berries

Servings: 1

Prep Time: 5 minutes

Total Time: 5 minutes

Ingredients:

- 1 cup Greek yogurt
- 1/2 cup mixed berries (such as blueberries, raspberries, and strawberries)

Instructions:

1. Spoon Greek yogurt into a bowl.
2. Top with mixed berries.

Tips and Variations:

1. Drizzle with honey or maple syrup for added sweetness.
2. Sprinkle with granola or chia seeds for extra crunch and nutrients.

Nutritional Information (per serving): Calories: 180 Protein: 20g, Fat: 1g, Cholesterol: 10mg, Carbohydrates: 20g, Fiber: 2g, Sugar: 15g, Sodium: 65mg

Apple Slices with Almond Butter

Servings: 1

Prep Time: 5 minutes

Total Time: 5 minutes

Ingredients:

-   1 apple, cored and sliced
-   2 tablespoons almond butter

Instructions:

1. Spread almond butter evenly over each apple slice.
2. Serve immediately or pack for a snack on the go.

Tips and Variations:

1. Sprinkle cinnamon on the apple slices before adding almond butter for a flavor boost.
2. Use peanut or cashew butter as an alternative to almond butter.

Nutritional Information (per serving): Calories: 280
Protein: 8g, Fat: 18g, Saturated Fat: 2g, Cholesterol: 0mg
Carbohydrates: 28g, Fiber: 6g, Sugar: 20g, Sodium: 2mg

Carrot and Celery Sticks with Hummus

Servings: 2

Prep Time: 10 minutes

Total Time: 10 minutes

Ingredients:

- 2 carrots, peeled and cut into sticks
- 2 celery stalks, cut into sticks
- 1/2 cup hummus

Instructions:

1. Arrange carrot and celery sticks on a plate or in a serving dish.
2. Place hummus in a small bowl and serve alongside the vegetable sticks for dipping.

Tips and Variations:

1. Add other vegetables like bell pepper strips or cucumber slices for more variety.
2. Flavor the hummus with additional ingredients like roasted garlic or red pepper for extra zest.

Nutritional Information (per serving): Calories: 150

Protein: 6g, Fat: 8g, Saturated Fat: 1g, Cholesterol: 0mg

Carbohydrates: 16g, Fiber: 4g, Sugar: 4g, Sodium: 300mg

Cottage Cheese with Sliced Peaches

Servings: 1

Prep Time: 5 minutes

Total Time: 5 minutes

Ingredients:

- 1 cup cottage cheese
- 1/2 cup sliced peaches (fresh or canned in natural juice)

Instructions:

1. Place cottage cheese in a serving bowl.
2. Top with sliced peaches.
3. Serve immediately, or chill in the refrigerator before serving for enhanced flavor.

Tips and Variations:

1. Sprinkle with cinnamon or nutmeg for a spice twist.

2. Substitute peaches with other fruits like berries, pears, or pineapple for variety.

Nutritional Information (per serving): Calories: 200
Protein: 15g, Fat: 5g, Saturated Fat: 2g, Cholesterol: 20mg
Carbohydrates: 20g, Fiber: 2g, Sugar: 18g, Sodium: 500mg

Whole Grain Crackers with Avocado Spread

Servings: 2
Prep Time: 5 minutes
Total Time: 5 minutes

Ingredients:

- 10 whole grain crackers
- 1 ripe avocado, mashed
- Juice of 1/2 lime
- Salt and pepper, to taste

Instructions:

1. In a small bowl, mash the avocado with lime juice, salt, and pepper until smooth.

2. Spread the avocado mixture evenly over the whole grain crackers.

3. Serve immediately to maintain the freshness and crunch of the crackers.

Tips and Variations:

1. Top with tomato slices or radish for extra flavor and crunch.

2. Sprinkle with chili flakes or add a few drops of hot sauce for a spicy kick.

Nutritional Information (per serving): Calories: 250
Protein: 4g, Fat: 15g, Saturated Fat: 2g, Cholesterol: 0mg
Carbohydrates: 27g, Fiber: 7g, Sugar: 2g, Sodium: 200mg

Baked Kale Chips

Servings: 2

Prep Time: 10 minutes

Cook Time: 10 minutes

Total Time: 20 minutes

Ingredients:

- 1 bunch kale, washed and torn into bite-sized pieces
- 1 tablespoon olive oil
- Salt, to taste

Instructions:

1. Preheat oven to 350°F (175°C).
2. In a large bowl, toss kale pieces with olive oil and salt until evenly coated.
3. Spread kale on a baking sheet in a single layer.
4. Bake in the preheated oven for about 10 minutes, or until the edges are brown but not burnt.
5. Serve immediately for best texture.

Tips and Variations:

1. Sprinkle with nutritional yeast before baking for a cheesy flavor.

2. Add garlic powder or smoked paprika for extra seasoning.

Nutritional Information (per serving): Calories: 150
Protein: 5g, Fat: 7g, Saturated Fat: 1g, Cholesterol: 0mg
Carbohydrates: 18g, Fiber: 3g, Sugar: 0g, Sodium: 200mg

Edamame with Sea Salt

Servings: 2
Prep Time: 2 minutes
Cook Time: 5 minutes
Total Time: 7 minutes

Ingredients:

- 2 cups edamame (fresh or frozen)
- Sea salt, to taste

Instructions:

1. If using frozen edamame, thaw under running water.
2. Bring a pot of water to a boil and add edamame.
3. Cook for about 5 minutes, or until fully heated and tender.
4. Drain and sprinkle with sea salt.
5. Serve warm or chilled.

Tips and Variations:

1. Toss with a splash of soy sauce or sesame oil for an Asian twist.
2. Sprinkle with chili flakes for added heat.

Nutritional Information (per serving): Calories: 120
Protein: 12g, Fat: 5g, Saturated Fat: 0.5g, Cholesterol: 0mg
Carbohydrates: 9g, Fiber: 5g, Sugar: 2g, Sodium: 120mg

Dark Chocolate (at least 70% cocoa) and a Handful of Berries

Servings: 2

Prep Time: 2 minutes

Total Time: 2 minutes

Ingredients:

- 2 ounces dark chocolate (70% cocoa or higher)
- 1/2 cup mixed berries (such as blueberries, raspberries, and blackberries)

Instructions:

1. Break the dark chocolate into small pieces.
2. Serve the chocolate pieces alongside the mixed berries.

Tips and Variations:

1. For a richer experience, melt the dark chocolate and dip the berries into it.
2. Add a sprinkle of sea salt or chili flakes to the dark chocolate for a flavor contrast.

Nutritional Information (per serving): Calories: 150
Protein: 2g, Fat: 9g, Saturated Fat: 5g, Cholesterol: 0mg
Carbohydrates: 17g, Fiber: 3g, Sugar: 12g, Sodium: 0mg

Rice Cakes Topped with Ricotta and Honey

Servings: 2

Prep Time: 5 minutes

Total Time: 5 minutes

Ingredients:

- 2 rice cakes
- 1/2 cup ricotta cheese
- 2 teaspoons honey
- Optional: sprinkle of cinnamon or sliced almonds

Instructions:

1. Spread ricotta cheese evenly over each rice cake.
2. Drizzle honey over the ricotta.

3. If desired, sprinkle with cinnamon or top with sliced almonds.
4. Serve immediately for best texture.

Tips and Variations:
1. Replace honey with a low-calorie sweetener for a lighter version.
2. Add fresh fruit like sliced strawberries or banana for extra nutrients and flavor.

Nutritional Information (per serving): Calories: 200
Protein: 8g, Fat: 8g, Saturated Fat: 5g, Cholesterol: 20mg
Carbohydrates: 25g, Fiber: 1g, Sugar: 9g, Sodium: 85mg

SAMPLE 7 DAYS MEAL PLAN

Below is a sample meal plan from the list of recipes provided earlier:

Day 1:

- **Breakfast (8:00 am):** Overnight Oats with Chia Seeds, Berries, and Almonds
- **Lunch (12:00 pm):** Grilled Chicken Salad with Mixed Greens and Avocado
- **Dinner (6:00 pm):** Baked Cod with Lemon and Dill, served with Steamed Broccoli
- **Snack (3:00 pm):** Almonds and Walnuts Mix

Day 2:

- **Breakfast (8:00 am):** Spinach and Mushroom Omelet
- **Lunch (12:00 pm):** Quinoa and Black Bean Wrap with Salsa
- **Dinner (6:00 pm):** Grilled Salmon with Asparagus and Quinoa
- **Snack (3:00 pm):** Apple Slices with Almond Butter

Day 3:

- **Breakfast (8:00 am):** Greek Yogurt with Flaxseeds and Honey
- **Lunch (12:00 pm):** Turkey and Hummus Sandwich on Whole Grain Bread
- **Dinner (6:00 pm):** Lentil and Vegetable Stew
- **Snack (3:00 pm):** Carrot and Celery Sticks with Hummus

Day 4:

- **Breakfast (8:00 am):** Avocado Toast on Whole Grain Bread with Poached Egg
- **Lunch (12:00 pm):** Grilled Chicken and Vegetable Kabobs
- **Dinner (6:00 pm):** Roasted Chicken with Sweet Potatoes and Brussels Sprouts
- **Snack (3:00 pm):** Greek Yogurt with Mixed Berries

Day 5:

- **Breakfast (8:00 am):** Smoothie Bowl with Kale, Banana, and Peanut Butter
- **Lunch (12:00 pm):** Vegetarian Chili with Avocado and Cornbread
- **Dinner (6:00 pm):** Grilled Shrimp and Vegetable Kabobs
- **Snack (3:00 pm):** Whole Grain Crackers with Avocado Spread

Day 6:

- **Breakfast (8:00 am):** Whole Grain Pancakes with Fresh Berries
- **Lunch (12:00 pm):** Stuffed Bell Peppers with Ground Chicken and Vegetables
- **Dinner (6:00 pm):** Beef Stir-fry with Bell Peppers and Brown Rice
- **Snack (3:00 pm):** Rice Cakes Topped with Ricotta and Honey

Day 7:

- **Breakfast (8:00 am):** Protein Smoothie with Spinach, Blueberry, and Yogurt
- **Lunch (12:00 pm):** Grilled Chicken and Quinoa Bowl with Roasted Vegetables
- **Dinner (6:00 pm):** Baked Sweet Potato Hash with Eggs, Turkey Sausage, and Bell Peppers
- **Snack (3:00 pm):** Dark Chocolate (at least 70% cocoa) and a Handful of Berries

Note: You can adjust the times to fit your schedule and preferences. Also, make sure to stay hydrated by drinking plenty of water throughout the day!

How To Implement this meal plan

Here's a suggested plan for implementing the recipes in the stages of cortisol detox:

Stage 1: Elimination (Days 1-3)

- Focus on removing processed foods and added sugars from your diet
- Incorporate stress-reducing techniques like meditation and deep breathing
- Start with gentle exercise like yoga or walking

Recipes to focus on:

- **Breakfast:** Overnight Oats with Chia Seeds, Berries, and Almonds (Day 1), Greek Yogurt with Flaxseeds and Honey (Day 2)
- **Lunch:** Grilled Chicken Salad with Mixed Greens and Avocado (Day 1), Quinoa and Black Bean Wrap with Salsa (Day 2)
- **Dinner:** Baked Cod with Lemon and Dill, served with Steamed Broccoli (Day 1), Lentil and Vegetable Stew (Day 2)

- **Snacks:** Almonds and Walnuts Mix (Day 1), Apple Slices with Almond Butter (Day 2), Carrot and Celery Sticks with Hummus (Day 3)

Stage 2: Transformation (Days 4-6)

- Introduce more protein sources like lean meats and fish
- Increase fiber intake with fruits, vegetables, and whole grains
- Incorporate more intense exercise like weightlifting and cardio

Recipes to focus on:

- **Breakfast:** Avocado Toast on Whole Grain Bread with Poached Egg (Day 4), Smoothie Bowl with Kale, Banana, and Peanut Butter (Day 5)
- **Lunch:** Grilled Chicken and Vegetable Kabobs (Day 4), Vegetarian Chili with Avocado and Cornbread (Day 5)
- **Dinner:** Grilled Salmon with Asparagus and Quinoa (Day 4), Roasted Chicken with Sweet Potatoes and Brussels Sprouts (Day 5)
- **Snacks:** Greek Yogurt with Mixed Berries (Day 4), Whole Grain Crackers with Avocado Spread (Day

5), Rice Cakes Topped with Ricotta and Honey (Day 6)

Stage 3: Optimization (Day 7 and beyond)

- Continue to focus on whole, nutrient-dense foods
- Incorporate adaptogenic herbs like ashwagandha and rhodiola
- Gradually increase exercise intensity and duration

Recipes to focus on:

- **Breakfast:** Protein Smoothie with Spinach, Blueberry, and Yogurt (Day 7), Whole Grain Pancakes with Fresh Berries (Day 8)
- **Lunch:** Grilled Chicken and Quinoa Bowl with Roasted Vegetables (Day 7), Stuffed Bell Peppers with Ground Chicken and Vegetables (Day 8)
- **Dinner:** Baked Sweet Potato Hash with Eggs, Turkey Sausage, and Bell Peppers (Day 7), Beef Stir-fry with Bell Peppers and Brown Rice (Day 8)
- **Snacks:** Dark Chocolate (at least 70% cocoa) and a Handful of Berries (Day 7), Greek Yogurt with Mixed Berries (Day 8)

SUPPLEMENTS AND HERBS FOR EFFECTIVE CORTISOL MANAGEMENT

Managing cortisol levels can be effectively supported with the help of dietary supplements and herbal remedies. These can complement a well-rounded diet and lifestyle adjustments aimed at reducing stress. This chapter provides guidance on integrating supplements safely and explores the benefits of various herbal remedies.

Integrating Supplements

When considering supplements, it is crucial to approach this as a complement to, not a replacement for, healthy eating and lifestyle habits. Always consult with a healthcare provider before starting any new supplement, especially if you have underlying health conditions or are taking medications, to avoid potential interactions.

Steps to Integrate Supplements:

Assessment: Evaluate your current health needs and goals.

Research: Choose high-quality, evidence-based products.

Monitoring: Keep track of your intake and any changes in your symptoms.

Adjustment: Review the effectiveness and adjust dosages as necessary, with professional guidance.

Supplements That Support Cortisol Management

Here's a list of supplements known for their ability to help regulate cortisol levels, along with recommended intake and timing:

Phosphatidylserine: Known for lowering cortisol levels induced by stress and improving athletic performance by reducing muscle damage.

- **Recommended Intake:** 100-300 mg per day
- **Timing:** Before bedtime or after exercise

Ashwagandha: An adaptogen that helps manage stress and reduce cortisol levels.

- **Recommended Intake:** 300-500 mg of a root extract per day
- **Timing:** Split between morning and late afternoon

Rhodiola Rosea: Another adaptogen effective in increasing resistance to stress.

- **Recommended Intake:** 200-400 mg per day
- **Timing:** In the morning or early afternoon, to avoid potential interference with sleep

Magnesium: Helps reduce cortisol levels, supports sleep quality, and assists muscle relaxation.

- **Recommended Intake:** 200-400 mg per day
- **Timing:** Before bedtime to help with sleep

Omega-3 Fatty Acids (EPA and DHA): Reduce inflammation and help lower cortisol levels.

- **Recommended Intake:** 1,000-2,000 mg per day
- **Timing:** With meals to improve absorption

Vitamin C: Can lower cortisol and support adrenal function.

- **Recommended Intake:** 500-1,000 mg per day
- **Timing:** With meals to enhance absorption and reduce stomach upset

B-Complex Vitamins: Support energy levels and reduce stress.

- **Recommended Intake:** Follow label recommendations as potency varies
- **Timing:** In the morning to support daytime energy levels

Herbal Remedies and Their Benefits

In addition to dietary supplements, certain herbs can be used to help manage cortisol and stress:

1. **Holy Basil (Tulsi):** Helps lower blood sugar, protect against infection, and ease joint pain, besides reducing stress and balancing cortisol.
   - **How to Use:** Often consumed as tea or supplement.

2. **Licorice Root**: Extends the half-life of cortisol, which can help in adrenal fatigue, though it should be used cautiously, especially in those with high blood pressure.
   - **How to Use:** As tea or a supplement. DGL (Deglycyrrhizinated Licorice) is a safer form for long-term use.

3. **Ginseng:** Renowned for its ability to improve stress adaptation.
   - **How to Use:** As a tea, extract, or supplement, typically taken in the morning to avoid interference with sleep.

4. **Lemon Balm:** Known for its calming effects, it can help reduce cortisol and alleviate anxiety.
   - **How to Use:** Often consumed as tea or in capsules.

5. **Valerian Root:** Helps improve sleep and reduce anxiety, indirectly aiding cortisol management.
   - **How to Use:** As a capsule or tincture, typically before bedtime.

NOTES

While supplements and herbs can significantly aid in managing cortisol levels, they should complement an already healthy lifestyle. Always discuss any new supplement with a healthcare provider, particularly if you have existing health issues or are on other medications. By carefully selecting and properly timing these supplements and herbs, you can enhance your body's ability to manage stress and maintain healthier cortisol levels.

LIFESTYLE MODIFICATIONS FOR STRESS REDUCTION

Importance of Sleep in Cortisol Regulation

Sleep is a fundamental aspect of health that affects almost every type of tissue and system in the body – from the brain to the heart, and even the regulation of important hormones like cortisol. Understanding the interplay between sleep and cortisol is crucial for anyone looking to manage stress and maintain overall health effectively.

Sleep and Cortisol: The Connection

Cortisol, known as the "stress hormone," follows a diurnal rhythm, meaning it fluctuates throughout the day. Levels peak in the early morning, helping to promote alertness and wakefulness, and taper off in the evening, facilitating relaxation and sleepiness. Disruptions in sleep can lead to altered cortisol levels, which not only impairs your ability to sleep but can also create a cycle of stress and hormonal imbalance.

1. **Cortisol Awakening Response**: This refers to a rapid increase in cortisol levels within the first 30 minutes after waking. Research shows that a healthy cortisol awakening response is linked to good sleep quality, suggesting that better sleep can enhance your body's ability to regulate cortisol naturally.

2. **Cortisol and Insomnia**: Elevated nighttime cortisol levels have been linked to insomnia, one of the most common sleep disorders. High cortisol can make it difficult to fall asleep or stay asleep, leading to a host of negative health effects associated with sleep deprivation.

Impact of Poor Sleep on Cortisol and Health

Lack of adequate sleep can cause higher and more prolonged levels of cortisol in the evening, which not only disrupts future sleep patterns but also contributes to:

- **Weight Gain**: High cortisol levels increase appetite and cravings for high-calorie foods.

- **Immune Dysfunction**: Chronic high cortisol weakens the immune system, making you more susceptible to infections.
- **Increased Anxiety and Depression**: Sleep deprivation exacerbates mood disorders, partially through its effects on cortisol and other stress hormones.
- **Cognitive Impairment**: Cortisol interferes with memory and concentration, and prolonged exposure can damage neurons in the brain.

Strategies for Improving Sleep to Regulate Cortisol

Improving sleep quality and duration can be one of the most effective ways to normalize cortisol levels. Here are some strategies that can help:

1. **Consistent Sleep Schedule**: Go to bed and wake up at the same time every day, even on weekends. This consistency helps regulate your body's internal clock and can help maintain your cortisol levels.
2. **Optimize Your Sleep Environment**: Make your bedroom conducive to sleep – cool, quiet, and dark.

Invest in a good quality mattress and pillows to support a comfortable night's sleep.

3. **Wind-Down Routine**: Develop a pre-sleep routine to help signal your body it's time to wind down. This might include reading a book, taking a warm bath, or practicing relaxation exercises such as deep breathing or meditation.

4. **Limit Exposure to Screens**: The blue light emitted by screens can interfere with melatonin production, a hormone that regulates sleep-wake cycles. Try to avoid screens at least an hour before bed or use blue light filters.

5. **Mind Your Diet**: Avoid caffeine and heavy meals close to bedtime. Instead, opt for a light snack that won't disrupt your sleep, such as a small bowl of whole-grain cereal with milk or a banana.

6. **Consider Sleep Aids**: If lifestyle changes aren't enough, consider speaking to a healthcare provider about temporary use of sleep aids. These should be used responsibly and as a last resort, as they do not solve underlying problems causing sleep disruption.

By prioritizing sleep and addressing issues that interfere with a good night's rest, you can effectively help regulate your cortisol levels, thereby reducing stress and enhancing your overall health and well-being.

Exercise and Its Effects on Cortisol

Physical activity is a powerful tool in managing stress and regulating cortisol, the body's primary stress hormone. While exercise inherently stimulates cortisol production temporarily, it also plays a crucial role in maintaining a healthy cortisol balance over the long term. Understanding how different types of exercise impact cortisol can help you tailor your physical activity routine to better manage stress and optimize your overall health.

Acute Effects of Exercise on Cortisol

During exercise, the body perceives physical activity as a type of stress, triggering an increase in cortisol production. This immediate rise in cortisol serves several important functions:

- **Energy Regulation**: Cortisol helps mobilize glucose, fatty acids, and amino acids to provide energy to working muscles.
- **Anti-Inflammatory Response**: Although cortisol is elevated during and immediately after exercise, this is followed by a reduction in inflammation as cortisol works to control the immune response triggered by exercise-induced muscle damage.

This spike in cortisol due to acute exercise is generally transient and should not be a concern unless the exercise is very high intensity or prolonged, as can happen with overtraining.

Chronic Effects of Regular Exercise on Cortisol

Engaging in regular physical activity has several long-term effects on cortisol dynamics:

- **Enhanced Resilience to Stress**: Regular exercise improves the efficiency of the cardiovascular, nervous, and endocrine systems. This enhanced fitness level allows the body to handle physical stress more efficiently, resulting in a more moderated cortisol response when faced with stressors.

- **Improved Cortisol Regulation**: Consistent exercise helps to normalize cortisol patterns, particularly helping to maintain lower and more stable levels throughout the day. This can contribute to better sleep cycles, mood regulation, and overall health.

- **Reduction in Cortisol Levels**: Over time, regular moderate exercise can help reduce baseline levels of cortisol in the body. This reduction is especially beneficial for those experiencing chronic stress or elevated cortisol levels.

Optimal Exercise Strategies for Cortisol Regulation

To maximize the benefits of exercise on cortisol levels, consider the following strategies:

- **Moderate Exercise**: Engaging in moderate-intensity exercise, such as brisk walking, cycling, or swimming for 30 minutes most days of the week, can help manage cortisol levels effectively without causing excessive stress on the body.

- **High-Intensity Interval Training (HIIT)**: While high-intensity exercise can temporarily spike cortisol levels, incorporating adequate rest and recovery, as well as keeping HIIT sessions short and infrequent (e.g., 2-3 times a week), ensures that the overall impact balances cortisol positively.

- **Strength Training**: In addition to aerobic exercises, strength training is important for overall health and can help improve the body's metabolism and response to stress. Aim for 2-3 sessions per week, focusing on major muscle groups.

- **Yoga and Mindfulness-Based Exercises**: Practices such as yoga and Tai Chi not only provide physical benefits but also incorporate breathing and meditation elements that significantly reduce stress and can help lower cortisol levels.

- **Adequate Recovery**: Allowing sufficient time for rest and recovery between intense workouts is crucial. Overtraining can lead to a sustained increase in cortisol, which may negate the benefits of exercise on stress and health.

Balancing Activity and Recovery

It's important to balance your exercise routine with your overall health and cortisol levels. Listening to your body and adjusting your exercise intensity and duration based on factors like stress levels, sleep quality, and general health can help maintain an optimal cortisol balance.

Regular, balanced exercise routines confer numerous health benefits, including more regulated cortisol levels, improved stress resilience, and better overall health. By choosing the right type and amount of exercise, you can harness these benefits effectively.

Creating a Stress-Reducing Routine for Effective Cortisol Management

Managing stress effectively is crucial for maintaining healthy cortisol levels and improving overall wellness. Developing a daily routine focused on stress reduction can help you manage cortisol, enhance your mood, and increase your energy levels. Here's how to establish a stress-reducing routine that fits into your lifestyle and helps you stay balanced.

1. Identify Stressors

Begin by identifying the sources of stress in your life. This might include work deadlines, relationship issues, financial pressures, or health concerns. Understanding what triggers your stress is the first step in managing it effectively.

2. Set Clear Boundaries

Once you know your stressors, set boundaries to help manage them. This might involve saying no to additional responsibilities, limiting work hours, or establishing clear rules for how others treat you. Protecting your time and emotional energy is key to stress management.

3. Incorporate Regular Physical Activity

Exercise is a powerful stress reliever. It can increase endorphins, improve mood, and, as previously discussed, help regulate cortisol levels. Incorporate activities you enjoy, such as walking, yoga, cycling, or team sports, into your daily routine. Aim for at least 30 minutes of moderate exercise most days of the week.

4. Practice Mindfulness and Meditation

Mindfulness and meditation can significantly reduce stress and lower cortisol levels. Spend 10-20 minutes a day practicing mindfulness or meditation. You can use guided sessions from apps or YouTube, or simply spend time in quiet reflection, focusing on your breath and being present in the moment.

5. Develop Healthy Sleep Habits

Sleep is crucial for cortisol regulation. Develop a bedtime routine that helps you wind down and signal to your body that it's time to sleep. This could include reading, taking a warm bath, or practicing gentle yoga or meditation. Aim for 7-9 hours of quality sleep per night.

6. Nourish Your Body with Healthy Foods

What you eat has a direct impact on how you feel and on your cortisol levels. Incorporate a diet rich in whole foods, lean proteins, healthy fats, and antioxidants. Avoid or limit caffeine and sugar, which can spike cortisol and increase stress.

7. Stay Connected

Social support is vital for managing stress. Stay connected with friends and family who uplift and support you. Sharing your thoughts and feelings can help you feel less alone and more able to cope with stress.

8. Schedule Regular Breaks

During the workday, take short breaks to step away from your desk or work environment. A brief change of scenery can help clear your mind and lower your stress levels. Try a five-minute stretching routine, a quick walk around the block, or a moment to sit quietly and breathe deeply.

9. Learn to Prioritize and Delegate

Assess your to-do list and prioritize tasks based on importance and urgency. Don't hesitate to delegate responsibilities when possible to reduce your workload and minimize stress.

10. Practice Gratitude

End each day by reflecting on what you are grateful for. Keeping a gratitude journal can shift your focus from stressors to what enriches your life, fostering a sense of contentment and reducing stress.

11. Seek Professional Help

If stress becomes overwhelming or leads to anxiety or depression, consider seeking help from a mental health professional. Therapy can provide strategies and support for managing stress effectively.

By incorporating these strategies into a daily routine, you can create a sustainable way of managing stress that minimizes the impact of cortisol on your health. Remember, the goal is to find what works best for you and adapt these practices to fit your unique needs and lifestyle.

OVERCOMING COMMON CHALLENGES

Embarking on a journey to manage cortisol and detox from stress is a significant commitment that can encounter various challenges. This chapter provides strategies for handling setbacks and stressful events, staying motivated throughout your detox plan, and adapting the plan to fit your evolving lifestyle.

Handling Setbacks and Stressful Events

1. Accept and Anticipate Setbacks: Recognize that setbacks are a normal part of any change process. Anticipate them and plan your response. When you accept that challenges will occur, you can approach them with a mindset that is focused on learning and resilience.

2. Develop Coping Strategies: Prepare a list of effective coping strategies that you can turn to during stressful times. This might include deep breathing exercises, talking to a friend, journaling, or engaging in a physical activity. Having a toolkit can help you manage stress without derailing your detox plan.

3. Reflect and Learn: After experiencing a setback, take time to reflect on what happened. Identify the triggers and think about how you can better handle similar situations in the future. Learning from each experience can strengthen your ability to manage future challenges.

4. Seek Support: Don't hesitate to reach out to others for help. Whether it's family, friends, or professionals like a therapist or a coach, support can make a significant difference in overcoming setbacks.

Staying Motivated During the Detox Plan

1. Set Clear, Achievable Goals: Break your detox plan into small, manageable goals. Celebrate each milestone to keep motivation high. Setting and achieving immediate short-term goals can build confidence and reinforce your commitment to the longer-term changes.

2. Keep a Progress Journal: Document your journey, noting not just what you eat and how much you exercise, but also how you feel physically and emotionally. Reviewing your progress can boost your motivation and help you see the tangible benefits of your efforts.

3. Visualize Success: Spend time visualizing your success. This mental rehearsal can enhance your motivation and help you stay focused on your goals. Imagine how you will feel and what your life will look like once you have achieved your objectives.

4. Adapt Incentives: Reward yourself for sticking to your plan. Choose rewards that do not contradict your detox goals (e.g., a massage, a new book, or a day trip).

Adapting the Plan to Your Changing Lifestyle

1. Be Flexible: Life changes, and so should your detox plan. Be prepared to adapt your strategies to fit changing circumstances—whether it's a change in your work schedule, family commitments, or social activities.

2. Incorporate New Habits Gradually: As your lifestyle changes, introduce new habits slowly so they can sustainably integrate into your life. This gradual approach helps prevent overwhelm and makes it easier to maintain these changes long-term.

3. Reevaluate Regularly: Periodically review your plan to ensure it still fits your needs and goals. This regular assessment allows you to make necessary adjustments and keep the plan relevant and effective.

4. Educate Yourself Continuously: Keep learning about stress management and healthy living. The more informed you are, the better equipped you'll be to make decisions that support your cortisol detox efforts.

5. Use Technology: Leverage apps and online resources to stay on track. Many tools can help you monitor your diet, exercise, and stress levels, providing useful feedback and reminders to keep you aligned with your detox plan.

By understanding and implementing these strategies, you can effectively navigate the challenges that come with managing cortisol levels and maintaining a stress detox plan. Remember, the key to success is persistence, flexibility, and a positive outlook.

MONITORING YOUR PROGRESS

Successfully managing cortisol levels through a detox plan requires ongoing assessment and adjustments. This chapter explores various tools and techniques to monitor your stress and cortisol levels, highlights when it might be necessary to seek professional help, and discusses how to adjust your diet plan based on the feedback from these evaluations.

Tools and Techniques to Track Your Stress and Cortisol Levels

1. Journaling: Keep a daily log of your stress levels, dietary habits, sleep patterns, physical activity, and any symptoms you experience. Note any correlations between changes in your routine and your stress or mood fluctuations. This can help you identify triggers and effective coping strategies.

2. Wearable Technology: Devices like fitness trackers and smartwatches can monitor your heart rate variability (HRV), sleep quality, and activity levels—indicators that can be influenced by cortisol. Some devices even offer features designed to monitor stress levels directly.

3. Apps for Stress Management: Several apps provide guided meditation, breathing exercises, and other stress-reduction techniques. These can be used to help manage daily stress and monitor changes in your stress levels over time.

4. Salivary Cortisol Test Kits: These kits allow you to collect saliva at home and send it to a lab for cortisol analysis. Testing your cortisol at different times of the day can help assess your cortisol rhythm, which should naturally peak in the morning and taper off by night.

5. Professional Health Monitoring: Regular check-ups with a healthcare provider who can order cortisol tests, such as blood or urine tests, to provide a more comprehensive view of your cortisol levels and adrenal function.

When to Seek Professional Help

1. Symptoms Persist or Worsen: If you've been following your detox plan but continue to experience high stress, fatigue, insomnia, or other health issues related to elevated cortisol levels, it's important to consult with a healthcare professional.

2. Mental Health Concerns: If you notice symptoms of depression, anxiety, or other mental health issues becoming prevalent, professional help from a mental health counselor or psychologist can be crucial.

3. Physical Health Changes: Unexplained symptoms like weight gain, high blood pressure, or persistent digestive issues warrant a visit to your doctor.

4. Guidance on Supplements and Diet Adjustments: Before making significant changes to your supplement regimen or if your dietary adjustments are not yielding results, seeking advice from a dietitian or a healthcare provider is recommended.

Adjusting the Diet Plan Based on Feedback

1. Analyze Your Journal: Look for patterns or changes in how you feel based on your dietary choices. If certain foods consistently correlate with higher stress or poor sleep, consider reducing or eliminating them from your diet.

2. Listen to Your Body: Your body's reactions can provide direct feedback. For instance, if you notice increased energy levels or improved mood after incorporating certain foods, these are positive signs that your dietary choices are beneficial.

3. Be Responsive to Change: As your body adapts to the detox plan, your needs may change. What worked initially might become less effective over time, requiring adjustments to portions, meal timing, or specific nutrients.

4. Regular Review with a Professional: Having periodic reviews with a dietitian or nutritionist can help ensure your diet continues to meet your nutritional needs and health goals, based on professional assessment and latest health data.

5. Experiment with Moderation: Sometimes, small adjustments rather than complete elimination can be effective. For example, instead of completely cutting out caffeine, you might limit intake to the morning hours to mitigate its impact on sleep.

Monitoring and adjusting your cortisol detox plan are key components of managing stress and maintaining overall wellness. By using the right tools, seeking help when needed, and being willing to make necessary changes, you can effectively navigate your journey toward better health.

Nothing Good Comes Easy So

Keep Showing up

MINDFULNESS AND EMOTIONAL WELL-BEING

In the quest to manage cortisol levels and improve overall health, mindfulness and emotional well-being play critical roles. This chapter explores cognitive behavioral techniques for managing anxiety, the benefits of journaling and other reflective practices, and how mindfulness can help maintain hormonal balance.

Cognitive Behavioral Techniques to Manage Anxiety

Cognitive Behavioral Therapy (CBT) is a widely used approach that helps individuals manage anxiety by changing negative thought patterns and behaviors. Here are some key CBT techniques:

1. **Thought Challenging**: This involves identifying and challenging the negative thoughts that contribute to anxiety. By questioning the evidence for these thoughts, evaluating their usefulness, and testing out the reality of negative predictions,

individuals can develop more balanced and less distressing thoughts.

2. **Behavioral Experiments**: Contrast your expectations of a particular situation with what actually happens. This can reduce fear over time and help you learn that what you fear often does not happen.

3. **Mindfulness-Based Cognitive Therapy (MBCT)**: This combines mindfulness practices such as meditation and breathing exercises with cognitive therapy. The focus is on becoming aware of all incoming thoughts and feelings and accepting them, but not attaching or reacting to them.

4. **Exposure Therapy**: Gradually, and in a controlled way, expose yourself to the situations that trigger your anxiety. Over time, this can reduce the power these triggers have over you.

5. **Relaxation Techniques**: Techniques such as deep breathing, progressive muscle relaxation, or guided imagery can help alleviate physical symptoms of stress and anxiety.

Journaling and Other Reflective Practices

Reflective practices like journaling can be powerful tools for emotional processing and stress management:

1. **Journaling**: Writing down thoughts and feelings can help clarify them and provide an opportunity for positive self-talk. It can also serve as a release mechanism, often leading to a reduction in anxiety and stress.

2. **Gratitude Journaling**: Daily writing about things for which you're grateful can shift your focus from stressors to positive elements of your life, enhancing emotional well-being.

3. **Mood Tracking**: Keeping a mood diary can help identify triggers for stress and patterns in mood fluctuations. This insight can be invaluable for managing emotional responses and planning effective coping strategies.

4. **Reflective Meditation**: Engage in meditation that focuses on introspection and the contemplation of specific questions or themes, promoting a deeper understanding of one's thoughts and feelings.

The Role of Mindfulness in Hormonal Balance

Mindfulness meditation has been shown to significantly impact physiological processes that influence hormones, including cortisol:

1. **Reducing Stress**: Regular mindfulness practice can lower cortisol levels by reducing stress and promoting a state of relaxation.
2. **Enhancing Emotional Regulation**: By increasing awareness of the present moment and decreasing reactivity to mental content, mindfulness can improve emotional regulation, leading to less emotional stress and lower cortisol spikes.
3. **Improving Sleep Quality**: Mindfulness and meditation improve sleep patterns, which is crucial for regulating cortisol and other hormones.
4. **Increasing Resilience**: Regular mindfulness practice can increase psychological resilience, making you better equipped to handle stress in a balanced way, thus maintaining healthier cortisol levels.

CONCLUSION

As we reach the conclusion of "The Cortisol Detox Diet Plan: A Step-by-Step Guide to Regaining Control Over Stress, Anxiety, and Hormonal Imbalances," it's important to reflect on the journey we've undertaken together. This guide has provided a comprehensive approach to understanding and managing cortisol through diet, lifestyle adjustments, and mindfulness practices. Each chapter has been crafted to equip you with the tools needed to reduce high cortisol levels and enhance your overall well-being.

Recap of Benefits and Outcomes

The Cortisol Detox Diet Plan offers multiple benefits that can lead to a healthier, more balanced life:

1. **Improved Stress Management**: By incorporating foods rich in nutrients that help modulate cortisol and adopting stress-reduction techniques, you are better equipped to handle life's challenges with resilience.

2. **Enhanced Sleep Quality**: Adjusting your diet and routine to include habits that promote good sleep can dramatically improve your sleep quality, which in turn helps regulate cortisol production.

3. **Boosted Energy and Mood**: With stable cortisol levels and reduced stress, you're likely to experience more consistent energy throughout the day and an improved overall mood.

4. **Hormonal Balance**: The dietary and lifestyle changes recommended in this plan help maintain optimal hormonal balance, contributing to better health and reduced risk of chronic diseases.

5. **Empowerment Over Your Health**: Learning to control your cortisol levels can empower you to take charge of your health, leading to long-term benefits and a greater sense of agency over your well-being.

Embarking on this detox plan requires commitment and persistence, but the rewards are well worth the effort. You now have the knowledge and tools at your disposal to make meaningful changes that can last a lifetime. Remember, managing cortisol and reducing stress is not a one-time task but an ongoing journey.

As you move forward, continue to adapt the principles and strategies outlined in this book to suit your evolving needs and circumstances. Stay curious and open to learning more about your body and its response to various stressors. Don't hesitate to revisit the sections of this book as needed, and consider consulting healthcare professionals to tailor the approaches specifically for you.

Finally, be patient and kind to yourself throughout this process. Change doesn't happen overnight, and there will be ups and downs. However, by consistently applying the lessons learned from the Cortisol Detox Diet Plan, you are on your way to a healthier, more balanced, and fulfilling life.

Thank you for allowing this guide to be a part of your journey to wellness. May you continue to grow stronger and more resilient, empowered by the knowledge that you have the tools to manage your stress and enhance your health. Here's to living a life with balanced cortisol levels—a life filled with peace, health, and happiness.

Health is wealth

Made in the USA
Las Vegas, NV
17 June 2024

91165035R00089